Brooke Jennings writes with a compelling realism that demands change. This heart-rending account compels the reader to turn on the light of truth and watch the culprits scatter like the cockroaches they are. Jennings, through Michael's horrendous ordeal, gives voice at last to those who have had no one to speak for them.

Amy Stark, M.E.D.

Living in a Place Called Beautiful is one of the most heartfelt books that I have read in a long time. Jennings is a warmhearted humanitarian that demonstrates a true love for her fellow man and gives a strong voice to the rights of anyone whose life has been changed by a disability. Through her book, she gives practical advice to anyone who will listen about what to avoid before accepting substandard care from nursing homes and other medical institutions. This book is a necessary read before making any decision concerning long-term care.

Mary Wright B.S. L.A.S.

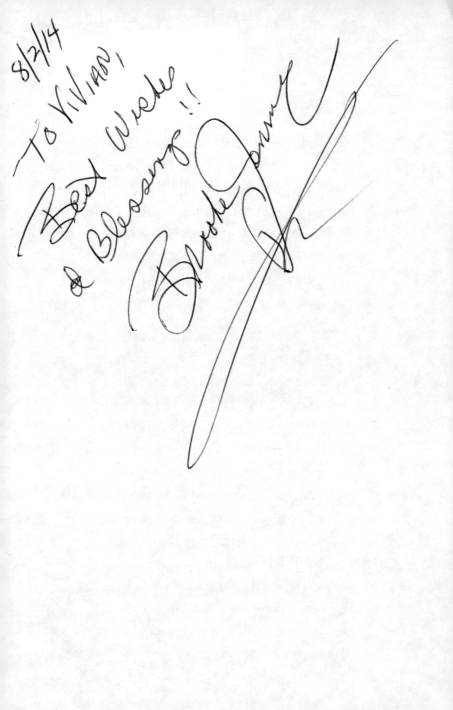

8/2/14
To Vivian,
Best Wishes
& Blessings !!

Living in a Place Called

Beautiful

Living in a Place Called

Beautiful

{ A Story of *Abuse* and *Death* in Healthcare }

Brooke Jennings

Tate Publishing & *Enterprises*

Published by Tate Publishing & Enterprises, LLC
127 E. Trade Center Terrace | Mustang, Oklahoma 73064 USA
1.888.361.9473 | www.tatepublishing.com

Tate Publishing is committed to excellence in the publishing industry. The company reflects the philosophy established by the founders, based on Psalm 68:11,
"The Lord gave the word and great was the company of those who published it."

Book design copyright © 2009 by Tate Publishing, LLC. All rights reserved.
Cover design by Brandon Wood
Interior design by Steven Jeffrey

Published in the United States of America

ISBN: 978-1-60247-756-8
1. Health Care: Abuse
2. Inspirational
09.03.10

DEDICATION

To Michael, a bright-shining star, who throughout his illness sent a message full of strength and courage. He became living proof that "angels come in all shapes and sizes," by giving more to those who knew him than he ever took away when he left.

To Janette, Christopher, grandchildren, and great-grandchildren: I leave you this book as a legacy and a gentle reminder that *life is short* and that the best time to love someone is when they are here with you, not after they are gone.

ACKNOWLEDGMENTS

I acknowledge my creative writing professor, Sue Hart, for her selfless work in helping me produce this book. Thanks to her valuable suggestions and expertise, this story has been brought to its current status.

I would also like to extend my deepest gratitude to Amy, a true friend who possesses a deep understanding and compassion toward anyone who has suffered from any form of adversity and who has helped me immensely to bring this book into existence. Lastly, I want to send a special thanks to my husband and best friend, Bruce, who has shown a tremendous amount of support and encouragement while I struggled with the production of this book.

FOREWORD

This compelling and, at times, heartbreaking story tells of Brooke Jennings' attempts to care for and protect her handicapped son. Sadly, she was unable to save him from the very people we believe we can depend on in the circumstances she describes.

Living in a Place Called Beautiful: A Story of Abuse and Death in Healthcare is not only a tribute to a beloved son, but a guide for readers who might be seeking long-term care for family members in nursing homes and other institutions. This is not an easy book to read emotionally, but it just might provide you with important information you will not find elsewhere.

–Sue Hart, Professor of English

One day Peter and John went up together to the temple at the hour of prayer, the ninth hour. And a certain man lame from his mother's womb was carried, whom they laid daily at the gate of the temple which is called beautiful, to ask alms from those who entered the temple; who, seeing Peter and John about to go into the temple, asked for alms, And fixing his eyes on him, with John, Peter said, "Look at us." So he gave them his attention, expecting to receive something from them. Then Peter said, "Silver and Gold I do not have, but what I do have I give you; In the name of Jesus Christ of Nazareth, rise up and walk." And he took him by the right hand and lifted him up, and immediately his feet and ankle bones received strength. So he, leaping up, stood and walked and entered the temple with them-walking, leaping, and praising God.

Acts 3: 1-8, NKJV

DISCLAIMER

All occurrences and conversations in this book were based on personal observations and recollections of the parties involved. In some instances, inner thoughts and dialogue have been recreated in an effort to portray the events depicted in the book. However, other events are as close to the exact memories as the sources permit. Many of the locations and the main characters' real names were changed. Some minor character's names were changed or omitted to protect the privacy of several individuals connected to this story.

TABLE OF CONTENTS

Preface

No parent ever expects to outlive his or her own child. Regardless of the circumstances, this type of loss can make their lives seem unbearable as they struggle to live each day without their sons or daughters.

Although I knew deep in my heart that I was not responsible for Michael's death, many of my days were spent reliving the painful memory associated with losing him. That was until I had the good fortune of crossing paths with a Jewish Rabbi. He was visiting his family in Idaho and was good friends with Bob Abrams, the private investigator investigating our wrongful death claim. Rabbi Stigler was a man who possessed a warm spirit and a compassionate nature. He listened with great intent while I spoke about Michael and the people responsible for harming him.

Although many years have passed since our initial meeting, I can still remember his keen insight, and his kind words have never been far from my thoughts.

"Brooke, whenever a parent loses a child, they receive a gift. Once you discover what Michael's passing has given you, you will be able to move on with a joyful heart."

Before meeting Rabbi Stigler, I was afraid that I would not be able to adequately portray my son's life or show the magnitude of his courage throughout his ordeal. However, I eventually realized that Michael's death had nothing to do with my intelligence, profession, or anything about me personally. It happened because of a flawed system that had already existed for many years. In fact, the system called *healthcare* had already been extending inadequate care to anyone who had the misfortune of crossing paths with it prior to my having too rely on it. Armed with this poignant and simple truth, I knew how important it was for our family to share the *gifts* we were given with the millions of people who will read this book.

INTRODUCTION

Whenever medical emergencies arise, most individuals do not possess the nursing skills needed to provide twenty-four-hour care to their family members. Consequentially, nursing homes and group homes have become the first source they turn to whenever a parent or spouse becomes terminally ill or incapacitated.

Because employers seldom offer their employees the option of health care insurance, patients are often forced to apply for assistance from charitable organizations and the medical community to help pay for their unexpected medical expenses. Despite their efforts to avoid any additional financial hardships, many of these applications will be denied due to limited services and long waiting lists.

Although family members want to provide emotional support to their loved ones whenever they become ill, it can still be difficult to find caregivers qualified to provide the emergency care needed. Consequentially, nursing homes and institutions have become a popular alternative to in-home care. Although most states do not require group homes to employ specialized nursing staff within the home, Medicare and Medicaid have agreed to allow severely impaired and mentally challenged individuals into these facilities, placing them at high risk for injury and death.

Once released, some prisons have made verbal and written agreements with large corporations to employ persons on probation and parole. As a result, people convicted of serious crimes have found a new line of work, and they are flooding health care's gates. Some have become certified nursing assistants (CNAs), physical therapists, and respiratory techs. Thanks to large corporations utilizing their efforts to employ the cheapest labor they can find, the medical community is becoming the criminals' playground. By ignoring their histories, medical facilities have enabled parolees to access to all kinds of goodies, such as patient medications, items of personal value, and victims.

Due to federally mandated programs, many professional organizations have become "felon friendly," and they are currently receiving tax reductions and free insurance policies in exchange for hiring newly released parolees.

Almost daily, somewhere across the nation, there are stories about medical workers who were found guilty of assault, rape, theft of medications, and murder. Although it can be argued that some of these cases are isolated, it is still puzzling why this type of criminal activity has made it into any of our medical facilities. It also leaves room for us to question whether this form of violence has always existed or if it has just now become more prevalent because the media and patient advocates have finally decided that someone needs to pay closer attention to the disabled.

Thanks to television shows like America's Most Wanted, 20/20, and 60 Minutes, child-abuse issues are touched on almost daily, yet no one seems to have taken the incentive to investigate the day-to-day deaths of disabled children or elderly patients in many of our nursing homes and institutions.

Supporting the expectation that people who live in nursing homes are sitting in wheelchairs and are lined up in hallways waiting for death to take them home lessens the chance that anyone would even care that there has been an increase in abuse cases or deaths in many of these long-term facilities. Perhaps, if we were to take the time to investigate, we might find that *two factors* killed some of these patients: the abuse/neglect they received at the hands of their caregivers and money. Simply put, many of these corporate enterprises are no different than many other capitalistic entities operating in America today. They are providing a service as cheaply as they can.

Although some medical facilities continue to offer substandard care, insurance companies have welcomed the chance to insure them. This sends a clear message to the victims of abuse and their families that they support this negligent way of doing business.

Because of child victims and their families, recent legislation has passed laws ensuring that all employees who work in daycare facilities are fingerprinted, and some medical institutions have caught on by requiring background checks before issuing licenses to their health care workers. Fortunately for them, this makes it look as though they are at least trying to protect their patients. Still, if anyone turned on the light of truth in some of these somber organizations, they would be shocked to learn that many of the rules have been overlooked and ignored when hiring people with prior felonies or violent misdemeanors.

Sociologists often agree that crime increases when there is a lack of education, social structure, or substance abuse. That, in turn, results in violence, lack of empathy, and crime. If we believe this statement holds any element of truth, then why are we employing persons who have already demonstrated an inability to grasp the damaging effects their actions have on society? In addition, why do we trust them to care for frail patients while paying them a wage?

After reviewing Michael's life, it became clear that my experience was no different from many others when I sought twenty-four-hour care for him. Needing immediate assistance, I reached out in good faith, believing our health care system was safe, efficient, and reliable, along with the people in it. After my child was laid to rest, I had plenty of time to think about the reasons why he died and how our healthcare system had failed him.

CHAPTER ONE

APRIL SORROW

As I walked down the hallway to my son's room, my mind was filled with more questions than answers. *Who would want to harm Michael?* After all, he was a frail young man whose laughter and smiles were contagious.

After preparing Michael's body for transport to the coroner's office, Misty, a nursing assistant who cared for Michael prior to his passing, handed me two large bags, containing his personal effects.

"I am so sorry, Mrs. Jennings. If there is anything I can do, please do not hesitate to call."

Nodding slightly in acknowledgement, I thanked her for the kindness she had shown to our family.

Michael was the youngest member of our family and he had two older siblings, Patrick and Maggie. Patrick was a service writer in the automobile industry, and Maggie was a registered nurse who possessed a natural gift for healing the sick.

Although my intention was to phone my daughter immediately upon returning home, the days events had taken their toll. I had been sleeping for close to an hour before Patrick woke me. Since Maggie lived in California, Patrick suggested I phone the police to ask for their assistance.

Saddened by our loss, they offered their condolences and agreed to be with my daughter when she received the news about Michael's passing. Although I was grateful for their kindness, I had forgotten to tell them which brother had passed away. Upon hearing the dreadful news, Maggie assumed Patrick passed away, not Michael! After learning that it was her youngest brother, it was as though a thousand knives had pierced her soul. Since a large part of Maggie's identity died with Michael that day, she declined to practice nursing for several years. When asked why, she would say it was because she felt betrayed by her peers and confused about why someone who swore to preserve life would take the life of her disabled brother.

Eventually, Maggie called home to let us know that she was scheduled to arrive in Idaho later that evening. Although I had originally planned on going to the airport with Patrick, I stayed home waiting for the coroner's office to call. Because Michael had died suddenly and without good cause, state law dictated that an autopsy be performed. After learning that Michael's cause of death was drowning, I called Pete. Although our divorce had been amicable, it had been over fifteen years since we had last spoken.

When Michael was born, I was forced to endure a dangerous delivery procedure commonly referred to as a "double breech, face-up birth." Since Medicaid refused to pay for most of the medical bills, Pete was forced to declare bankruptcy. Angry and bitter, he refused to take an active role in Michael's life and seldom paid his child support. Although I was angry that Pete disregarded Michael, I knew deep in my heart that it was my obligation to inform him that our son had passed away. Anxious, I picked up the receiver and dialed his number.

Upon hearing my voice, Pete sensed that I was not calling to be social.

"Brooke, what's wrong?"

"Michael is dead!" I shouted.

Pete's reply came after a few moments pause. "Well, sweetie, it wasn't like we didn't know that this would happen one day."

"What did you say? He was murdered!" I screamed.

Pete's answer was anything but cordial. "Well, sweetie, if you're looking for any money, I don't have any."

Sickened by his remark, I began scolding Pete, telling him what a terrible father I thought he was for abandoning Michael. However, I never got to complete my tirade. He hung up the phone before I could finish.

Although I initially believed that Pete was saddened by his son's death, I also believed that he used the argument between us as an excuse not to come to the funeral or offer his condolences. Thirteen years later, I had the opportunity to speak with him about Michael's book. Somehow, I hoped he would explain why he never went to his son's funeral. However, five minutes into our conversation, he reinforced his thoughts about Michael's passing. "If you're looking for any money, I don't have any!"

After speaking with the coroner's office, Patrick and I tried to recall the details leading up to Michael's death. Since he had always been wheelchair-bound, Patrick and I felt that it was impossible for him to die from drowning unless foul play was involved.

CHAPTER TWO

THE GIFT

After living in private Catholic schools during most of my childhood, I chose not to participate in any regimented religious services as an adult. However, when Michael was born, I placed my personal feelings aside and had him baptized in the Catholic church. Consequentially, since Michael expired on Good Friday, the church would not allow him to be buried until the following Monday.

The cemetery chosen as Michael's final resting place was picturesque and was located in one of the older sections of town. The gravesite was nestled securely between several large spruce trees on top of a hill. Standing alone, I took a few moments to reflect on our tragedy.

This is it, I thought, the final resting place for my son.

The day of the funeral was typical for early spring, and it had been raining for several hours before we arrived at the cemetery. As I stood by Michael's casket for the final time, the rhythm of the rain beating on its roof stirred something deep inside of me. It was the realization that I would never be able to hold him, kiss him, or enjoy the sound of his laughter. Fighting desperately to maintain my composure, I began to imagine the feeling of his face against my cheek whenever I read him bedtime stories. Nursery rhymes were his favorite, and we often found ourselves laughing until we cried whenever I sang and our fingers danced to the tune of the "Itsy Bitsy Spider."

Once the funeral service concluded, I remained at Michael's grave for several minutes. Overtaken with grief, I became filled with a desperate need to know that whatever dimension of time he was forced to dwell in, he was happy.

"Michael," I whispered, "please give me a sign. Show me that you are happy. Please!"

Since Michael was taken from our family so suddenly, it made me question my role as a mother, my sanity, and my beliefs in God. No matter how I tried, I could not understand what I had done to deserve this sort of punishment. Of course, over time I learned that losing my youngest child was never intended to be a punishment. In fact, as strange as it might sound, Michael's death was a gift.

Although a large part of my belief stemmed from being his mother, I was also influenced by an incident that happened a few days after Michael's birth.

Following a traumatic entrance into the world, Michael contracted sepsis, a severe bacterial infection, and within two weeks he passed away. Since he had been confined to an incubator from the moment he was born, I was not allowed to hold him or feed him for the entire two weeks following his birth.

I do not recall how long I held Michael after he passed away, but eventually I was approached by an elderly woman who believed in the "laying on of hands." Of course, being raised as a Catholic, I did not necessarily believe in the practice, but Minnie never showed any concern that I was a nonbeliever. She just smiled sweetly and asked for permission to pray for Michael.

When the prayer service ended, Minnie returned to the waiting room, while I stayed in Michael's room, waiting for a sign that God had heard our prayers.

While Pete and I prepared to leave the hospital, one of the nurses who had been caring for Michael came running into the hallway. She was frantic as she waved her arms, shouting, "Wait! Don't go! He's alive! He's alive!"

Thanks to Minnie and her courage to trust in God's mercy, Michael made a full recovery, and within days of receiving such a wonderful miracle, I traveled to New York and shared my experiences with my father, Don. He, along with other family members, listened intently when I spoke about

Michael's miracle healing. Since all my family members were Catholic, they were not comfortable with accepting any rituals outside of the Catholic faith and they emphasized how they would never accept anything as foolish as the "laying on of hands." Within time, Don also conformed to the family's wishes, and he ordered me to stop attending healing services. When I refused his demands, he became so angry; he told friends that I had "snapped." He also insisted that I leave his home until I could come to my senses.

Pete had enough of the healing services too. Although he never attended any of the services, he started calling me names like "Bible Thumper" and "Holy Roller." Years later, he would say he could not handle having a handicapped child and a wife who went to church regularly. He needed more and started drinking, going to strip clubs, and having extra-marital affairs. The final blow came when he announced that he was leaving our family for a teenage girl hired to babysit Michael.

CHAPTER THREE

FIGHTING THE SYSTEM

By 1979, Pete and I had been divorced for two years. Occasionally, we shared a phone call and spoke about Michael, but the guilt and the financial scars left over from our bankruptcy caused him to remain angry and bitter. Once our divorce was finalized, he refused to pay his child support, forcing me to depend solely on community services to get the help our son needed.

Since cerebral palsy is caused from damage to the motor area of the brain, Michael was spastic and needed patterning classes. During the school year, the public school he attended covered those expenses, along with supplying his speech classes and physical therapy. However, as Michael grew older, it became harder for me to support many of his day-to-day needs without working two jobs.

When Patrick and Maggie were in elementary school, most of our days began by six in the morning. Typically, I would usher the children off to school before going to work, and their babysitter would supervise them until I arrived home around six in the evening.

Although several years have gone by, I can still remember a story that helps to explain how difficult it was for a single parent to raise a handicapped child during the early seventies. After leaving work, I had gone to pick up the children from the sitter. Normally, they could be found either running around the neighborhood or watching television in her living room. However, on this particular day they were not with the babysitter. They were in the custody of social services!

As the pieces of the story began to unfold, I learned that Maggie and Patrick had been left unattended when they went to our apartment to change into their play clothes. It was dark in the small two-bedroom dwelling, and Maggie had tried to open the blinds to let more light into her room. Because she pulled the string to the blinds out instead of down, they became unattached from their brackets and struck Patrick. After treating his injuries, the paramedics noticed that Michael was unable to sit up without assistance, and they filed a neglect report with DFS.

Dr. Lewis was our family pediatrician, and he was at the emergency room when the children arrived at the hospital. Since he was familiar with all of my children's medical histories, he spoke at great length with the social worker regarding Michael's disabilities. Although the workers' actions seemed impulsive, it is important to note that he was influenced by the early seventies paranoia about child abuse. Laws regarding spanking as a form of punishment were challenged, and people were becoming hyper-vigilant.

Prior to Michael's birth, children with similar medical conditions were considered an embarrassment for their families, and they were institutionalized and kept out of the public eye. Hence, by the time Michael was six years of age, DFS had visited our family on three separate occasions. Eventually, tired and strained from worry, I sent Michael to live in a rehabilitation center.

The facility was owned and operated by the Catholic church, and it was supported by public donations. It had thirty beds for children ages two and up, and Michael was allowed to live at the facility until he aged out at fourteen. Michael thrived during his stay at the center, and the sisters loved him as though he was their own. Living under their careful guidance made him happy, and he grew into a handsome young man who smiled and laughed continuously.

CHAPTER FOUR

THE SEPARATION

After living in Europe for two years, I returned home to attend my father's funeral. Once his estate was settled, I used my inheritance to purchase a restaurant in northern Virginia. Since the main gate to the military base was only three blocks away, it was customary for its personnel to take advantage of our lunch specials. Bob, a chief petty officer in the navy, ate lunch at Dominic's almost daily, and within time we met and fell in love. Our courtship lasted for about a year before we married, and other than the typical protest about sharing their mother, the children adjusted well to their new family life. Since my husband had considered the military his home, he was referred to as a *lifer*. However, once we were married, we knew that Bob could be sent to a new duty station at any time.

The California coastline was breathtaking, and the weather was comparable to the Massachusetts shoreline during the summer. Shortly after arriving in Southern California, we enrolled the children into a public school and purchased a new home. Like most teens, Patrick and Maggie were occupied with making new friends and engaged in extracurricular activities at school. Bob and I took advantage of our free time by painting our new home and landscaping its backyard. Our hope was that the project would be completed sometime before summer's end.

Although there were the usual delays, our project was close to its completion when Bob became ill from asthma attacks. At first, his doctors believed that he suffered from allergies, and they scheduled weekly breathing treatments, hoping to ease his symptoms. However, once he was diagnosed with high blood pressure and panic attacks, the navy considered Bob "unfit for duty." Although the military offered Bob shore duty in Virginia, he opted to accept a medical discharge, and, as his health continued to spiral out of control, his depression became a large concern.

At fifteen, Patrick was a normal outgoing teen who usually committed normal teenage offenses. Failing to take out the trash was one of his largest indiscretions, and it frustrated my husband to no end. Normally, whenever Patrick failed to complete his chores, he would receive a lecture and lose part of his allowance. However, on this particular occasion Bob became so outraged by his son's lack of responsibility, he threw the garbage into his bedroom. Maggie was at home the day Bob exploded, and when she inquired as to why he would do such a "stupid" thing, he assaulted her.

After reporting the abuse, the police chose not to file charges. Since Bob was on active duty and subject to double jeopardy if arrested, they decided it would be best to release him into my custody with the understanding that he would seek immediate medical attention. Because he was enlisted, the military had strict rules about their personnel making appointments to see civilian physicians. Unfortunately, before an appointment could be scheduled on the base, Bob assaulted Patrick.

Along with the separation came many other changes. Because my household income was drastically reduced, the children and I had to move into a smaller house. I also quit my city police job to work for the federal government. Although the pay was not as lucrative, the position gave me the opportunity to teach at one of their police academies and pass on my experience to other men and women in law enforcement.

By the beginning of 1989, military bases across the country were closed, forcing many of the federal police officers who had five or more years of government service to scramble for key positions in other states. Although I was new to federal service, I was fortunate enough to be offered a position on a naval base located in Virginia.

Since I had lived in Norfolk in the past, I was

not concerned about moving back east. Rather, I was worried about the three-year waiting period that was required to get Michael into a rehab center—the chance of having to leave him behind in California. After receiving a welcome letter from the command, they requested that I fly to Virginia in order to complete the physical agility testing. Under normal circumstances, this would have been good news, but at that point I had not made any concrete plans regarding Michael's care.

Anyone who has ever traveled with a severely disabled individual knows firsthand that it is not an easy task. You need help and lots of it. At age fourteen, Michael was unable to sit up unassisted, and he was getting heavier to lift with each passing day. Flying him to Virginia on an airplane made a lot more sense than driving in a car for five days, but I could not afford to fly to Virginia and then drive across the country with all of our belongings. Although I hated the idea of leaving him with strangers, I decided to admit him into a temporary group home until I could start my new job and arrange for his day care.

After meeting with an organization that specialized in handling medical care for children with disabilities, I arranged for Michael to be placed into a group home. The facility was used as a transition house where children often stayed until other arrangements could be made for in-home care, and they had several children from military families at the facility.

It was owned and operated by an elderly couple who claimed to have taken care of many special-needs children, and after touring the home, it appeared adequate to handle Michael's twenty-four-hour needs. Convinced that he would be in safe hands, I agreed to a ninety-day placement.

CHAPTER FIVE

THE DECEPTION

After accepting an official offer of employment with the military police and moving back to Virginia, the budget was cut, forcing the government to place a freeze on hiring. What had originally promised to be a great opportunity and fresh start quickly turned sour for Michael and me.

After securing a part-time job at a local restaurant in Virginia Beach, I notified the Wades that Michael's short-term placement was going to become a lengthier stay.

Although I had been working six shifts per week, there was not enough money to pay for Michael's trip home following the initial ninety days, so I took on a second job cooking at a local steakhouse. I also answered an ad for a roommate to share expenses. By midsummer, I was confident that Michael would be home before Christmas, and I rented a three-bedroom home to accommodate his needs. I also agreed to work overtime at the restaurant during weekends. It was my usual Saturday shift, and I had arrived early to help train a new server who had no experience with waitressing or restaurant operations. Unbeknownst to me, my attempts at making the additional money needed to bring Michael home by Christmas would prove to be a costly mistake.

Initially, I had no idea that I had suffered any trauma when the kitchen door struck my arm, but within a week I learned my elbow was broken. Terrified at the possibility of becoming unemployed, I called Bob, pleading for help. He sent me twenty-five dollars.

As the New Year rolled in, I was more determined than ever to make the best of my situation, so I began looking for a job outside of the restaurant business. Eventually, my efforts paid off when I found a cashier's position at a small grocery store. Since my car had been repossessed for lack of payment, I was in desperate need of transportation. Eventually, I found an older Toyota Corolla that needed a paint job. It was primer grey and belonged to an elderly gentleman who, due to health problems, was unable to continue driving. He was not interested in making a large sum of money from its sale, and after a quick road test, I returned home with my new purchase.

As much as I tried to convince myself that I was making progress, the reality of my situation revealed that I was not any closer to getting Michael home than I had been six months earlier. Weary from my failed efforts, I made a conscious decision to quit my job and move back to California. Although I knew that another move could ultimately delay Michael's return home, I was mentally drained and emotionally exhausted from trying to think of other alternatives.

Within hours of deciding to leave Virginia, I received a phone call from a social worker. A new medical facility had opened its doors, and they were interested in accepting Michael as a patient. The facility was classified as a hospital/institution, and they had three beds available for patients with disabilities. After touring the facility, I learned that they had a pediatrician on staff who specialized in caring for handicapped children.

Along with the typical physical therapy and speech classes, it offered the residents additional activities, such as movie nights, outings to the mall, and weekly trips to the park and movies.

Originally, I had no interest in placing Michael in an institution since they usually housed mental patients and adults. However, this hospital housed those kinds of patients in a different wing, making it safer for everyone concerned. Visitations were liberal, and the staff encouraged full involvement with your child. The children who were school age attended classes in-house and received one-on-one instruction. After filling out the initial application, the hospital accepted Michael on a tentative basis. Ecstatic, I busied myself making the necessary arrangements to bring him home.

CHAPTER SIX

MRS. WADE

After admitting Michael to the group home in Oregon, I entrusted Patrick and Maggie with watching over their younger sibling, and as far as I knew, Michael was perfectly fine and doing well. After receiving the good news about Michael's admission to Hampton Roads Rehabilitation Center, the final plans for his return home were nearing completion. I was finally beginning to feel that a difficult patch in my life was ending when the other shoe dropped. It was a late fall evening when Patrick called with the disturbing news. He was distraught and believed that Michael's life was in mortal danger.

After hearing how the group home denied Patrick visitations with his brother, I contacted East Side Regional and the Wades. Although both agencies assured me it was a simple case of "miscommunication," I was not comfortable with their explanations. Since Michael resided at a group home, Patrick should have been able to visit during normal business hours, yet Mrs. Wade insisted that he always came to visit at an inopportune time. Common sense dictated that he might have visited his brother at an inconvenient time of day on one occasion, but not every time.

After speaking with Mrs. Wade, I became convinced that her story sounded suspicious and insincere. Fearing for Michael's well-being, I phoned the police and requested a welfare check for my son. After meeting at a predetermined place and time, Patrick and the police officers went to the group home. When they entered the facility, they found Michael isolated in a rear bedroom, far removed from human contact. Closer examination revealed that my youngest child was laying face down, covered in urine and feces.

When the police first saw Michael, they were alarmed, but they did not know how to treat the complaint. Somehow, Mrs. Wade's gentle manner convinced them that Michael had always been thin and had come to live with her in a malnourished state. She also stated that he was under a doctor's care and that everyone, including East Side Regional, knew he was not thriving.

Satisfied with Mrs. Wade's story, the police left my disabled child at the group home and in Mrs. Wade's care. Despite Patrick's protests, the police refused to listen to our concerns, calling it "a civil matter."

After several threats to have Mrs. Wade arrested,

she eventually relented and admitted that Michael had not adjusted well to his placement. She also conceded that part of the problem stemmed from not knowing how to feed my son. Following several failed attempts to have East Side Regional remove my son from her home, Mrs. Wade admitted to moving Michael into a bedroom located in the rear of her home and laying him on his stomach. Because Michael had poor motor control, he was unable to lift his head without assistance, and after three days he had chewed a dime-size hole in his bottom lip. It still sends a chill up and down my spine every time I think about the terror this child experienced because of the Wades.

After demanding to know why she would commit such a vile act, Wade stated, "I asked East Side Regional to remove your son from my home and they ignored me." Frustrated, she chose to lock Michael away until either he died from starvation or someone removed him from her residence. After hearing her sick confession, I phoned the police for the third time. However, they remained firm in their resolve by emphasizing that since my son was under a doctor's care, it was "out of their hands." They concluded by stating "if I you do not agree with how Wade is treating Michael, you can come here and remove him from her home, yourself." Furious by their lack of professionalism, I phoned East Side

Regional and demanded that they fly Michael to Virginia within the next twenty-four hours.

Despite the lack of cooperation, I filed a police report accusing the Wades and East Side Regional of child abuse. Unhappy over my refusal to dismiss the allegations of abuse, a police detective in charge of Michael's case made a special point of telling me how the district attorney's office would decide if it was abuse or not and "not to remain hopeful." Although I had witnessed many cases of child abuse during my career, nothing could have prepared me for what had been done to my child.

When Patrick arrived at the airport, Michael was slumped sideways in his wheelchair. His arms and legs were rigid, and he suffered from abnormal posturing. His eyes were fixed staring ahead as though looking into an empty void, and he did not seem to possess any recognition of his family. What was left of my normal, happy-go-lucky son with the contagious smile was nothing more than an empty shell. Since Michael's voice was almost nonexistent, he would emit low-pitched whimpers similar to a suffering animal.

Following a complete examination, doctors from the Children's Hospital in Norfolk released the details of my son's abuse. According to their reports, Michael had become so dehydrated that he suffered from baseball-size stools, anemia, dehydration, and malnutrition. Since he spent most of his days hungry and cold, he cried continuously. Frustrated from having to listen to his screams for help, Mrs. Wade forced this defenseless child to lay face down to muffle his cries. Because Michael had been denied water for several days, his tongue had become swollen and blistered, and it placed tremendous strain on his kidneys. His mouth was full of sores, and his head was infested with cradle cap.

Two months after Michael's initial rescue, his doctors were still performing surgeries to keep the blood supply flowing to his feet. Because of the beatings he had sustained to his face, he refused eat from a spoon and needed to have a feeding tube surgically placed into his stomach.

Several months passed before The Sentinel interviewed Mrs. Wade and revealed Michael's story. His horrific ordeal was published by a newspaper that was well-known for having strong political slants regarding health care issues. When the story aired, Mrs. Wade told reporters that she had abused Michael because she discovered that "he had suffered from cold sores and was afraid of becoming infected." She attempted to justify her actions by switching the blame to the school and East Side Regional, stating, "Everyone withheld that information. Had I known, Michael would not have been allowed into my home." Due to her ignorance and abusive actions, Mrs. Wade felt Michael would infect the other children. After separating him from the other residents, her husband fed him Ensure Plus and baby food, but barely enough to keep him alive.

Originally, when Michael went to live with the Wades, he was thin for a normal fourteen-year-old, but his weight was acceptable for his condition. When he left the Wades' home, he weighed sixty-three pounds.

While The Sentinel worked feverishly to find the underlying cause of Michael's abuse, one of the doctors who initially treated him for his malnourishment told reporters, "If the neglect and abuse had continued for another few days, Michael most likely would have died."

Years later, and only after Michael's lawyer deposed witnesses at his wrongful death hearing, he discovered that one of the possible causes for Mrs. Wade's neglectful behavior was the word "contagious" stamped in red ink across my son's school records. Unbeknownst to East Side Regional, the school nurse, paranoid about fever blisters placed a memo into his school files. It was addressed to the principal of Michael's grade school and it urged the school board to expel my son, because he was "contagious, posing a health risk whenever he displayed fever blisters." Cold sores never justified the abuse and neglect of my child, yet by all accounts, the Wades were allowed to remain in business until 1992. Over thirteen children remained in their custody and care following public allegations of abuse by our family. It was only after being sued and exposed by the news that they agreed to close their doors.

Two years after the initial allegations of abuse, a police investigator discovered that the Department of Family Services had received numerous reports about the neglect of other patients living in this group home, yet they deliberately turned a deaf ear and a blind eye to Michael's neglect in order to keep the doors of the facility open.

CHAPTER SEVEN

THE CODE OF SILENCE

Following several heartbreaking months of watching Michael suffer through several life-threatening surgeries, it was a relief to see him gain weight and his strength return. Pete was still living in Virginia when Michael was transferred to a rehab center, and he made every attempt to take an active role in our lives during this difficult time. He visited once or twice a month, but he did not offer any financial assistance. During Michael's hospital stay, I tried to visit him daily and on weekends. On my days off, I stayed busy writing to the authorities in Oregon about Michael's case, with very little success. In a last-ditch effort, I wrote to the governor and the mayor of the city. A separate letter, dated June 5, 1991, was written to the chief of police, regarding his officers and their lack of professionalism in handling Michael's case. The department heads within the police division did not respond for three months, and only after *The Sentinel* published another article about Michael's plight. Chief Fisher cited "miscommunication" as the reason for the delay. He also went on record stating how he attempted to seek charges against the Wades for the alleged abuse, but "neglect could not be established." The medical reports did back up my claims of abuse, and Chief Fisher affirmed, "Neglect was obvious, but the problem was that no one could establish that the act was willful."

In a memo to the papers, he wrote, "I feel that the great distance that separated us contributed greatly with us not being able to communicate more directly and often, and it tended to exacerbate your understandable frustration in this case." Before ending his letter, Chief Fisher added, "It does concern me that you feel you could have been better served, and I continually direct my commanders to look introspectively to improve what we do. I have already instructed my Investigation Bureau commander to see that these long-distance investigations are handled more personally to avoid any additional misunderstandings such as I feel arose in this case."

Although I knew the Wades had no malpractice insurance, I filed a civil action for $3.5 million dollars. It was not that I ever expected to receive anything close to resembling that amount, but I did want them out of business. Hitting them hard in their pockets was the only way I knew to get their attention and to send a message that they were not going to abuse my son, or any other child, and get away with it.

The Wades might have been skilled enough to get past local law enforcement, but I knew that no child could have been neglected and pushed to the brink of death unless it was "willful." With all of the experience and the number of years they claimed to have cared for children, how could the police chief possibly feel comfortable citing that the reason behind not prosecuting the Wades was based on something as ridiculous as "there was no proof that they were governed by will without regard to reason"?

Additional reports written by independent investigators revealed that DFS had received several complaints about this facility, supporting the argument that they chose to ignore the evidence placed in front of them. Whatever the reasons, everything strongly suggested that East Side and the State Board of Licensing deliberately ignored the warning signs. By the end of the investigation, I knew that if someone had taken the time to examine all of the prior allegations, Michael would have been spared the horrible neglect that had befallen him.

Redwood had always been a town filled with old money and a mega million-dollar tourist trade, and I am sure that the lack of interest in pursuing a criminal case in this matter was nothing more than a political move on the DA's part to avoid bad publicity for their thriving little town's industry. Buying a politician was easy there, and in Michael's case, I felt they were having a bargain sale.

Another roadblock encountered was the distance factor Chief Fisher mentioned. Since I was in Virginia trying to get a case prosecuted in Oregon, it was easy for the system to take advantage of our family by sweeping the case under the rug. Michael was helpless and completely dependent upon others for his survival, so to use the term "miscommunication" as a reason not to protect him was just another way of saying, "We screwed up, we don't care, and we are not going to fix it."

Another disconcerting factor was the investigating officers having been my mentors. I trained under their careful guidance and admired these people, respected them, and wanted to be like them. Proud to have taken an oath to protect and serve, I swore never to ignore injustice by refusing to go that extra mile and help those less fortunate than myself. When Chief Fischer blamed distance and miscommunication as a reason not to seek charges against the Wades, I felt he was just as guilty of harming Michael as the willful acts of the group home. Worst of all, I felt betrayed by a system I had grown to love, and I no longer believed the criminal justice system worked for the little people.

After collecting and examining all of the facts related to the case, it was clear that a double standard existed. Had I committed such a vile act, I would have been hooked, booked, and put away with the DA appearing on every local and national television show, bragging about how wisely his office was spending our tax dollars by helping to bring about justice. If Michael had been abused today, the entire nation would most likely be sending e-mails to every talk show host and news station, demanding that I receive life in prison without any possibility for parole. However, neither of those things happened to Mrs. Wade or anyone else connected to Michael's abuse. Our family was left to deal with the far-reaching effects that would eventually assist in killing Michael in 1995.

Prior to the civil trial, the head administrator for the State Disabilities Committee at the state capitol became outraged over the publicity Michael's case was receiving, and he sent a representative to address the issue. The meeting was at my attorney's office. Mistakenly, I assumed the representative was sent to help me get justice by addressing Michael's abuse, and I welcomed the chance to speak with him. However, this man spoke plainly, and within moments he informed everyone involved that he was not there to help Michael or our family. He was there to convince us that it would be in everyone's best interest to drop the entire fight. Politically, he explained, the case was becoming a nightmare for the State of Oregon, the governor, and the office of disabilities. The words, "We want you to stop talking to the media about this case," seemed to be a direct hint for everyone to keep quiet. I took its meaning to be a possible threat. Angry, I fired back in rebuttal. I argued that my son had been starved to the brink of death and someone needed to pay for his neglect. Unmoved by my demands for justice, the man's answer was to threaten me openly. He clearly stated that if I appeared for any type of hearing in any court, with the intention of suing for Michael's alleged neglect, the government would arrange for me to be arrested for threatening a government official. He even went on to say, he could care less about the whole case! When the meeting ended, it was clear that he wanted this entire incident to be swept under the carpet before thousands of parents appeared on the capitol steps, screaming for justice.

Although outraged by this man's direct threats and lack of concern for Michael, I have to admit that his attempts at intimidation worked. There was no way I could go to jail. Who would care for Michael? Seeing no way out, I yielded to the pressure and settled out of court.

Months later, I wrote a letter to Washington D.C., describing my son's neglect. I sent his medical file, the abuse report from the police department, and photos from The Sentinel to President Bush Sr. Within weeks, Washington responded by sending an official memo to Oregon asking for a full investigation into the alleged abuse. I am not sure what the outcome was regarding his case after the memo was received, or if anyone ever responded back to Washington. All I know is that I did everything possible to bring this issue out into the open and avoid any further legal problems for our family. Due to the distance factor cited by Chief Fisher, no charges were filed through the DA's office. In the end, the civil case initiated on Michael's behalf was settled out of court. After being beaten, starved, and left for dead and suffering through five life-threatening surgeries, Michael received a mere $1,300 for all of his pain and suffering.

CHAPTER EIGHT

COLORADO

After failing to get the needed support to prosecute the Wades, Michael and I moved to Colorado. After being openly threatened by a government official, it gave us a chance to put the horrible injustice behind us. After relocating, I applied for a job cooking at a nursing facility part-time. The hours were flexible, and my roommate babysat Michael. Despite the abuse he had endured in Oregon, he appeared happy and continued to keep a smile and a laughter that could take your cares away.

When it came to playing, Michael was just like any other boy. He enjoyed playing on the floor or having someone wrestle with him. Many of his responses were similar to other children his age, and sometimes it was difficult to remember that he had any mental disabilities whatsoever. One of the biggest problems for Michael was his inability to know the difference between playing and real danger; so he had to be guarded at all times. Stairs were a real concern, and he often became stuck under the coffee table or behind chairs. Although Michael's safety was always top priority, writing this story reminded me of an incident that was instrumental in making me question my ability to continue caring for him alone.

Although he attended special classes, Michael was subject to the same rules as the other students, and every year he had to have a school physical. By the time Michael entered eighth grade, he had recovered from most of the effects of his malnutrition and weighed well over ninety-five pounds. Although I would never have done anything to jeopardize my child's physical well-being, I attempted to carry Michael unassisted down a flight of stairs. My ill-timed decision was costly, and it ended with us both falling down the staircase. To this day, I do not know how I managed to hang on to my son as we tumbled, but it was a miracle that either one of us was not seriously injured. Michael, on the other hand, thought the entire experience was hysterical and laughed until he cried.

This accident was influential in convincing me that Michael should be placed into another rehabilitation center. However, after nearly losing his life at the Wade's group home, I feared that Michael's life would be placed in jeopardy. Torn between what was best for Michael and my own personal needs, I chose to look for a one-story apartment.

Despite my good intentions, many of the properties listed were either too expensive for my modest salary, or they did not have any handicapped accessible amenities. Other owners were afraid, if Michael got hurt on their properties, their insurance rates would have skyrocketed, and they too, refused to rent to us. Eventually, I decided that it was safer to concentrate my efforts on finding a rehab center for Michael than it was to care for him at home.

Past experience told me that trying to locate an adequate facility capable of handling Michael's twenty-four-hour needs was not going to be easy. However, I began my search by talking with the State Commission for Nursing Home Regulation and Safety. Usually, they can tell you if a particular home has had any serious violations placed against it and what services a nursing home offers. I also made an appointment to speak with the administrators at my place of employment. Through them, I learned Michael qualified to stay in a nursing home.

When Michael moved into Memorial Gardens, we celebrated his fifteenth birthday and prayed, believing all of the terrible things that our family had endured over the years had become part of the past. Finally, I felt comfortable enough to believe our family had gotten a break from the constant struggles connected to health care, lawsuits, and the medical issues common to raising a disabled child. However, this false sense of security did not last, and by the following year the Colorado Nursing Home Regulation Board dropped the other shoe by declaring, no child/person under the age of twenty-one could reside in a nursing home.

For our family, this new regulation meant that Michael had to either return home or move to group home. Frantic, I appealed the decision, and after six weeks we learned that we had won our appeal.

With every victory comes a price, and in this case it was asking the nursing facility to change their entire internal structure to accommodate Michael's needs. Of course, Memorial Gardens declined the request, and a week later we received a letter advising us that Michael had to move out. By the spring of 1993, DFS had forced me to place Michael in another group home. Because of the abuse in Oregon, I never felt comfortable about my child living away from my watchful eye, and this placement was no exception. Unfortunately, my back was against the wall, and I had no choice but to accept his placement. However, I would quickly learn that my instincts had nothing to do with past events when I received an emergency phone call from the hospital in Park City, Colorado. Once again, another group home had been negligent by breaking my son's femur. After being questioned about the injury, group home administrators offered five different versions of how his leg had been broken. Although the fracture was a spiral fracture, it is an uncommon injury and usually found in child abuse cases. Caused from a twisting motion, it can often lead to shock, blood loss, and death.

Once I was notified that the group home had lied about how Michael's injury occurred, I knew they were trying to cover their tracks. Wanting to protect Michael, I filed a police report and hired an attorney to represent him. Prepared to take whatever steps were necessary to ensure we would not have a repeat of the Oregon case, I promised myself there would be charges filed this time, followed by a prosecution.

Although I did everything I could to protect Michael, charges were never brought against the group home or anyone responsible for my son's injury. Doctors, who treated my son for his injuries, made it perfectly clear they were not going to state that the injury to his leg was a direct result of abuse, because they feared being sued. Another surgeon refused to set Michael's leg after learning he was on Medicaid! He justified his decision by stating, "It is a waste of time and money since he is never going to walk anyway."

Upset by my inability to protect my child, I believed I was having a meltdown. I also believed that no one cared about Michael and that my inability to get justice for him somehow made me a failure as a mother. When Michael's three-week hospital stay ended, his civil rights attorney filed a negligence suit. The case settled in 1994, and after attorney's fees and out-of-pocket expenses, Michael was financially able to purchase his own home.

When the doctors refused to fix Michael's broken femur, his leg became four inches shorter, and he suffered from chronic pain. Because Michael was forced to live a sedentary lifestyle following his injury, he began to experience recurring bouts of pneumonia. If he had any chance of remaining healthy and active, he would have to receive constant physical therapy. Wanting nothing but the very best for Michael, I allowed him to be transferred to a rehab center in New Mexico for three months.

CHAPTER NINE

NEW BEGINNINGS

While Michael was in New Mexico recuperating from his injuries, I had plenty of time to think about the abuse he sustained in Oregon and Colorado. If I was ever going to protect him, it was important for me to understand why the medical professionals who swore to protect him kept harming him. Months of research about the internal structure of nursing homes and group homes helped to explain why many of the things that happened to Michael were continuing to play out in his life. One of the biggest revelations came once I realized he had been mistreated simply because he could not speak up or defend himself from attack. This alone allowed him to become the poster child for exploitation, and it gave his caregivers a tremendous opportunity to steal the Medicaid monies provided to them by our government.

Another reality check for me was the labels that were assigned to him from birth by the professionals caring for him. Over the years, I have personally heard physicians use the terms, *vegetative state* and *poor quality of life* when dealing with disabled individuals. These labels have unconsciously given permission to health care workers to dismiss handicapped individuals as not being conscious enough to know what is happening to them. Many times it sends a mixed message and gives criminals and abusers the permission they need to pick these type of patients as their next victim.

Patients in group homes and other long-term facilities have been forced to depend on overworked and underpaid social workers to protect them. As a result, many social workers visit these homes once every ninety days and only after phoning the caregivers. If our health care systems allow them to continue operating in such a lax fashion, people like Michael will continue to fall through the cracks and ultimately die at the hands of strangers. If our healthcare system allows them to operate in such a lax fashion.

Armed with this new and startling information, I began to see that health care workers who abused patients were no different from the predators who roam the streets handpicking their victims prior to molesting them and killing them. The only difference I could find between street criminals and medical abusers was that one of them had the boldness to apply for a license.

While continuing the search for additional

reasons why our health care system had not been protecting Michael, the data became even more frightening. It seemed to suggest that over the last several decades there has been an increasing number of reports about handicapped individuals being mistreated. This indicates that it has become an epidemic of huge proportions. So why, as a society, have we ignored this problem? Could it be that the majority of administrators, nurses, and nursing assistants are afraid of lawsuits, criminal charges, or losing their jobs? If not, why have they chosen to remain silent?

Once the reality of what Michael had endured took root, I vowed to do whatever was necessary to ensure that he could never be subjected to this abuse again. On January 15, 1994, Michael returned home from the rehabilitation center in New Mexico, and he became a homeowner. This was a milestone for him, and for the first time in his life he had a chance of having the security and freedom to live in his own home.

After the closing on his new home. Michael and I stayed busy, purchasing the needed equipment for his care. We rented a hospital bed, a Hoyer lift (used for transferring patients to and from their bed), a shower chair, and a special recliner for the living room. Although, Medicaid provided his feeding tubes, pump and formula, everyday essentials were the sole responsibility of his family. Since he still had residual income from his neglect suit, he was required to either spend it or lose it, so we hired a contractor to build a handicap ramp and bought him a van to transport him back and forth to doctor's appointments.

Under normal conditions, Michael had enough energy for three people, but with all of the stress from moving he began running low-grade fevers, so I took him to the emergency room. Once admitted, Michael's doctor ordered a chest X-ray and blood work. Although he did not know the immediate reason for my son's fever, his instincts told him that whatever was making Michael sick had to be treated aggressively before it became serious.

Lab tests eventually confirmed that Michael had contracted a serious case of pneumonia and blood poisoning from living at the rehab facility in New Mexico. Since his condition was left untreated for several weeks, bacteria had entered through his feeding tube site, placing his life in grave danger. Because he was already at the hospital, his doctor ordered additional tests as a precautionary measure. Through those tests, we learned that Michael had also acquired a small leak surrounding his feeding tube opening in his abdominal wall, which was causing him to aspirate the contents of his food. From now on, the doctor cautioned, any time Michael was lying down or in bed, he had to remain at a thirty-degree angle to prevent any future risk of aspiration or death.

Having a handicapped child was demanding, and I knew that I could never return to work unless I had assistance caring for Michael. Idaho had a program that enabled disabled patients to receive care in the privacy of their own home though the Medicaid Waver Program, but it had a waiting list of one to five years. The benefits allowed $2,000 per month to be paid to a live-in caregiver, and the responsibility of finding one fell on to the family. Because I was Michael's mother, Medicaid refused to pay me to stay at home and care for him. Once again, it looked as though we were forced to have another stranger care for him. The only difference was, this time they would invade his home.

CHAPTER TEN

MICHAEL

When Michael was born, he was premature, weighing less than five pounds. Regardless of the challenges he faced throughout his life, he always remained a kind and gentle spirit that laughed continuously. He was never able to sit up or roll over on his own power, but he could scoot on the floor backwards and follow you from room to room, laughing and shouting with glee. To Michael, every moment was a new adventure.

By his first birthday, his doctors were concerned about his lack of coordination, and he could not hold his head up without assistance. Although he was intelligent and happy, many of the health care professionals that knew Michael never saw him as a person; they viewed him as a science project. They knew that there was nothing short of a miracle that could change his quality of life, and they often took the opportunity to express that he did not have one. Although many of the doctors who treated Michael were callous or insensitive, many of the specialists were kind and hopeful. By the time Michael reached his second birthday, cerebral palsy had become his official diagnosis, along with other labels like "vegetative state" and "disconnected."

In order to gain a better understanding of my son's disability, I began attending free seminars sponsored by the local children's hospital in Virginia. The lectures focused on infants who were born with cerebral palsy. Since little was known about this crippling disease, it was deceiving. Most of the time, Michael was very limited in his physical abilities, such as walking, talking, and rolling over, and he had to invent different ways to communicate his needs.

Watching television was a favorite pastime for Michael, and it was normal to see him enjoy Gilligan's Island and cartoons. Although Gilligan was one of his favorite television characters, the doctors were never encouraged whenever I shared how much Michael enjoyed watching comedy shows.

One time, I was visiting Michael at the hospital. Before entering his room, I stopped in the hallway, momentarily, to remove my coat. The television was on, and I could hear him laughing hysterically at Gilligan's antics. Directly across the hall was an elderly man who was watching the same show. Listening intently, I could hear both of them laughing at the same things and at the same time. This assured me that the doctors were mistaken about Michael not having a quality of life, especially after demonstrating that he could understand something as complex as humor.

When Michael became old enough to attend classes, he was enrolled in a public school. This was a big adjustment, especially since he could not be in a classroom with regular students. According to the teachers, the reason for this decision was that the schools were unable to answer his need for special equipment, time, and attention. Report cards were another problem for Michael. Even today, many of our grading processes are based on manual performance, and special needs children often fall short if they cannot meet the physical demands placed on them.

When Michael was in third grade, I took him to a school psychologist for an evaluation. Three-quarters of the testing was based solely on his ability to walk, sit, stand, pick up objects, and read aloud. Since he had always been in either in a wheelchair or on the floor scooting, physically he was very limited in what he could do. The psychologist administering the test asked Michael to stand up, pick up a spoon that she had placed on the floor, and hand it to her. Even though these were impossible tasks for my son, it was never taken into consideration. Because he was unable to meet the demands placed on him, he received zero points toward his final score. Disturbed by the results, I asked the school psychologist why there were no specific tests for disabled children. She explained that no other testing had been made available, and all handicapped individuals had to use the same grading system as people without disabilities. Unfortunately for Michael, intelligence testing was not as important as physical ability. When the testing ended, his test scores indicated that he was functioning at a six-month-old level. Shortly before his death, he was retested and found to be functioning at a three-year-old level. I am sure that part of this significant change came after he received glasses and could see what he had previously only been able to feel or hear. Because Michael had several years of public school under his belt, either one of these things could have become the catalyst that improved his social understanding.

Social retardation is a label the school often used to describe Michael and any other person or group of persons that responded differently in society because they we not exposed to normal social situations and stimuli like other students. At first, I was not offended when they called Michael socially retarded because it made sense that if you cannot see it, hear it, or feel it, you cannot learn it. At least you cannot learn it easily. This makes a person socially delayed. However, the term "socially retarded" seems to send a larger message that the person is also mentally disabled. and when used inappropriately, it can cause a person's physical limitations to become completely misunderstood. Many of these children are bright and more sensing than the average bear. They often develop natural abilities that we as higher-functioning adults ignore or deny. In hindsight, if we say mentally challenged children and adults are socially retarded, we show them disrespect and how ignorant we are. I have no doubt after living with Michael for nineteen years that he was just as smart as anyone else. He was just trapped in a body that did not function properly. When Michael was seven years old, he was just as active as other boys were his age. He loved music and anything that popped out and surprised you. Fisher-Price toys were some of his favorites, and whenever he finished playing, I would place the toys under his bed for easy access.

Living with a handicapped child enables a parent the privilege of seeing how they can create their own special ways of communicating their feelings and desires. A perfect example of this came after laying Michael down for a nap. I had taken advantage of the time to catch up on my sleep and decided to snooze. When I awoke, Michael was missing. Frantic, I ran room to room searching for my missing child. Unable to locate him, I stood quietly by his bedside, trying to imagine who could have stolen my child. Suddenly, I heard Michael break out in hysterical laughter. Somehow, he had managed to escape from his bed under his own power and, after dropping onto the floor, he scooted underneath his bed to play with his toys. Although I was relieved that he was safe, I was also amazed! It had always been stories such as these that made me doubt the doctors and what they were saying about Michael's disabilities. Mentally, he seemed fine. Physically, he was challenged, but doctors automatically believe that if something is broken physically, it is also broken mentally. Unfortunately, with this kind of limited thinking, the baby can often get thrown out with the bathwater.

Michael's world changed considerably when his femur was broken. He was no longer able to scoot from room to room, making any previous form of exercise obsolete. Losing his ability to move independently forced him pay closer attention to things on television and in his immediate environment, and I believe it encouraged him to become more in-tune to the things around him.

By 1989, Michael's life had become consistent. His time was divided evenly between school, home, and the hospital. Fevers of 101 degrees were common, and he usually had to have canisters of oxygen on hand to help him breathe. As his former lifestyle became obsolete, considerable amounts of my waking hours were spent worrying about Michael's overall health and future.

Although I had to spend a lot of time dealing

with all of Michael's medical needs, Patrick and Maggie continued to live far from home. Like most adults, they remained busy with their careers and raising families. Maggie called daily, and Patrick mostly called on holidays and special occasions.

Maggie lived in California for most of her adult life, and she had a completely different sense about family than Patrick. After attaining her nursing degree, she chose to remain home with her children until they graduated from junior high school. She also continued to stay close to her baby brother and me. Patrick, on the other hand, spent most of his teenage years living life in the fast lane. Fast women, fast cars, and a motto of "there is always tomorrow" dominated his family life and relationships. After high school, his relationship with Michael had fallen by the wayside, and for several years he chose not to remain close to his immediate family. Surprisingly, following the birth of his first child, Patrick did a complete turnaround and became and excellent father. Whenever you saw Patrick, you saw Patrick Jr. They were reflections of each other and thicker than thieves. It was clear to everyone that the sun rose and set on his firstborn child, and I have no doubt that he would have given his life to protect him. As Patrick entered into his early twenties, he renewed his commitment to Michael, and it became important for Patrick to make up for the years that he was away. Moving to Idaho with Michael and me would prove to be one of the most important decisions he ever made as a brother, a son, and as a man, and we were proud to have him back in the family.

Michael had been dead for eight years when Patrick called, crying. He spoke about how guilty he felt that he had not taken the time to develop a closer relationship with his family, especially his brother. Walks in the park seemed appealing now, and he wished there was some way to turn back the hands of time and start over...only it was too late. One of the most important members of our family was missing.

Patrick had only been living with us four months when his youngest sibling passed away. Although I knew he would never be able to make up for those lost years, the moments they shared were precious! I encouraged Patrick to hold on to those memories and to use them as a gentle reminder that, "life is short, and to remember that the time to love someone is when they are here with you, not after they are gone!" I knew that he could never make up for the lost years, but the moments they did share were precious. I encouraged him to hold on to those memories and to use them as a gentle reminder that life is short, and the time to love someone is when they are here with you, not after they are gone.

When Michael's life ended so tragically, it made me realize the unspeakable horrors he had suffered at a very young and tender age. In order to keep myself from sinking into despair after he died, I tried to focus on some of the positive things that happened to him while he was alive. One of my favorite memories was when he received his first pair of glasses. He was nineteen before science had developed any new form of eye testing for disabled children. Michael could not read an eye chart, so it was impossible for anyone to determine what his prescription should have been. When the doctor placed his glasses on his face for the first time, he drew in a long, deep breath and said, "Ah." Watching his expression helped me to realize that he had probably never seen anything except shadows or black and white blurred images throughout his life. My final memory of that glorious day was when Michael turned to me, laughing with glee, and uttered, "Ma."

Overcome with emotion, I hugged him and kissed him, all the while crying tears of joy. During follow-up visits, Michael's eye doctor explained that my son's vision was 20/750. Learning how blind he was helped me to understand why he had developed many of the habits he displayed. Now, I know beyond any doubt that he navigated through life by relying strictly on voice, touch, taste, and smell. It solved the mystery about why Michael always placed his toys on his nose whenever he played with them. They had to be that close in order for him to see them!

CHAPTER ELEVEN

MOM

Born in Raleigh, North Carolina, in the fall of 1950, I was the second of nine children. Father was a Merchant Marine stationed at Paris Island, South Carolina, and my mother, Jane, was only sixteen when she became a mother for the first time. Feeling tied down and overwhelmed by an abusive relationship, she returned to New York to live with her mother.

Grandmother was Romanian, and Grandfather was Italian. A butcher by trade, he spent sixteen hours per day working and trying to support his wife, daughter, and two young grandchildren. The apartment we lived in was a uninsulated four-room wooden shack built on stilts. It was located next to a cemetery and down the street from the college I would eventually attend.

Mechanicsville was an old mill town filled with long rows of old clothing stores and abandoned coat factories. The neighborhood was typical for the mid-fifties, and it was complimented by a mix of

Italian, Polish, and Irish immigrants living together and raising families, all in search of a better life. Whenever I walked down Main Street, past the long rows of weathered storefronts, aromas of homemade bread, sweet sausage, and soup filled the air.

Grandmother was a homemaker, and shortly after coming to live with her, our grandfather passed away. Forced to survive by whatever means necessary, our Grandmother supported herself by taking in laundry to wash. Still, the money was scarce, and Betty and I would race home from school, only to find that there was nothing to eat, forcing us to go to bed hungry and wanting. Neighbors, tired of our constant begging, contacted the Sisters of Charity. They arranged for us to live at a local orphanage. During our stay, I learned that an orange was something I could eat, and shoes were something I could wear to keep my feet warm during the winter.

Grandma, weary from trying to support Jane asked her to leave her home. Unable to find legitimate employment and keep up with the expenses from raising two small children, Jane became desperate. Unfortunately for us, her next decision would alter the course of our destinies forever. After abandoning my sister and me in a barn outside of Whitehall, New York, she ran away. Since foster homes were not available in the mid-fifties, disposing of two small children became a big problem for our mother, Jane. She was on the run from our father, and she thought that if she deposited us at the orphanage again, he would have to be notified. Frantic and alone, her quick drive into the country solved her dilemma. Hungry and scared, Betty and I snuggled close together deep within a large stack of hay. It was Ed Sutherland's barn, and it held an assortment of chickens, dairy cows, and, two small children, freshly abandoned by their mother.

Milking cows at 4:00 a.m. was a daily routine for Ed. The farmer was barely awake, still wiping the sleep from his eyes, when he saw two little blonde girls with big brown eyes staring back at him. Troubled, he swept us into his arms and took us to his wife, Judith. She fell in love with us from the start, accepting us as her own. She even wanted to adopt us, but the Sutherlands had six children of their own. Because of Ed's decision, not to adopt, Betty and I were passed from family to family until the Demur's and the Wilson's came along. Both families wanted children, so finding Betty and me was a blessing. The downside was, neither family wanted to adopt *two small* children from the same family.

Following a brief court appearance, Betty was sent to live with the Wilson family, and I with the Demur's. The Wilsons had one natural daughter of their own, unlike Don and Peggy who were childless. Normally, both parents were required to sign the adoption paperwork before anything could become final, but Jane was reluctant to offer any information about my father's whereabouts. By the time my adoption became final, I was seven years old.

Initially, when my father learned that Betty and I were offered up for adoption, he became angry. He also refused to sign any paperwork unless he was paid one thousand dollars for each of his children. Furious, the juvenile judge handling the proceeding threatened to have him jailed for extortion. Knowing that he was facing jail time and he would never receive any compensation, he displayed his contempt and arrogance for the entire court process by refusing to sign the adoption papers for Betty. When Grandmother learned that our mother had abandoned us, she tried to get us back from the authorities. When they refused to give her custody, she tried to have our mother prosecuted for neglect. However, no one had any interest in penalizing Jane for being desperate and poor. When the dust settled, our mother consented to our adoption in exchange for five hundred dollars from the Demurs and a bus ticket to Florida to watch the horse races.

As a teenager, I often cleaned houses to buy extra amenities like makeup and hair spray. Vale, a disabled neighbor, needed help with cleaning and laundry, so every weekend I would stop by and help her with chores. One weekend, I was at her home cleaning when a neighbor stopped by for a visit. Being a typical teen, I took the liberty of eavesdropping on their conversation. The visitor was inquiring if the Demurs had any plans of telling me that Betty and I were related. I was shocked! As far as I knew, Betty was just a neighborhood girl I chatted with at the bus stop each morning. Excited to learn that I had other family, I raced home to ask the Demurs if what I heard was true. Their response was not what I expected. I was grounded for asking the question, sent to my room, and forbidden to have any contact with Vale or Betty ever again.

Growing up in separate families was difficult, and it meant that Betty and I could never be together as a family. As I grew into a young adult, there were many times that I wanted to ask the Demurs about Betty and me, but their Italian heritage and proud belief system dictated that under no circumstances was anyone to know I was not their blood. As far as they were concerned, the adoption would always remain a private matter and dirty laundry. From day one, they made it clear: it was not open for discussion!

The schools I attended as a child, were private Catholic schools located in Watertown, New York. Don, my adoptive father, was a successful business-person who traveled extensively as a commercial Real Estate broker. Peggy, his wife, was an ex-model in the clothing business and who worked for Solomon Fur Company in the early 40's. She was also an alcoholic who resented him bringing home any little bundle of joy that was not her own. Life at the Demurs' home was anything but pleasant with their constant arguing over her drinking or his infidelity whenever he was away on business trips.

While I was growing up, a typical day for me consisted of school and chores. Weekends were spent cleaning, dusting or ironing. On Sundays, I was allowed to watch television for one hour, but I was seldom allowed to play outside, unless it was inside my own backyard. Neighborhood children often came by but were quickly turned away and discouraged to return. It did not take long for them to learn not to invite me to any birthday parties.

After graduating from high school in 1968, I still had not gone to a dance or a football game. My room literally became my prison, but in many ways it was my sanctuary. I learned to use it to hide myself from the physical and verbal attacks I often endured when Peggy became intoxicated. Finally, by age eighteen, I managed to get far away from the toxic influence of the Demurs, and within time I healed from my childhood wounds.

When Don passed away, it was twelve long years since I had first left New York. After returning for his funeral, it was clear my surrogate family was not going to go out of their way to make me feel welcomed. They took great pleasure in reminding me that I was not "their blood." Out of respect for Don, they agreed to be silent about their true feelings until his death. It never bothered me that they disagreed about my adoption; what bothered me was the dishonest way they had treated me as a child.

After being confronted so maliciously, it was as though a switch was thrown deep inside. It was difficult, but once the funeral service ended, I began to understand how far some people were willing to go to deceive another person. Thirty years was a long time to wait to crush another person's spirit. I can only imagine how difficult it must have been for them to tolerate a small, innocent child in their home, laughing with glee as she opened the Christmas presents they had so graciously bought for her.

Although growing up with the Demurs was difficult, I had many moments when I believed a guardian angel sat on my shoulder, and Don's funeral would prove to be no different. Since Don's sisters had chosen the funeral setting to begin their vicious attacks, they ended it by introducing me as "Don's adopted daughter, Brooke." Embarrassed and taken aback by their remarks, I quietly contemplated walking out and leaving the final arrangements completely on their shoulders.

At the end of the service, I was saying my good-byes to the last of the guests when I noticed two elderly nuns from St. Peter's Parish enter the room. I assumed the Monsignor had asked them to stop by and recite the rosary in honor of the dead. After stopping at the casket to pay their last respects, they approached me and asked if I was Brooke. At first, I did not recognize them, but after searching their faces, I realized they were my first- and eighth-grade teachers. Sister Agnes was the first to hug me and speak.

"We saw the death of your father in the paper, and we said, 'That's our little Brooke. She is in trouble and she needs us.' We are here Brooke, how can we help you?"

Throughout my life, I have always been blessed with little miracles like this to share. Because the sisters raised me while I attended school under their careful guidance, most of my memories about them have always been precious. Whenever the Demurs wounded my small, childlike spirit, the sisters mended it. Whenever they crushed my dreams, the sisters gave me new ones. In addition, when my relationship with the Demurs ended, the sisters showed me that love is not what you say, it is what you do, by renewing theirs. Just as they had demonstrated their love toward me as a child, they continued to love me unconditionally well into my adult years. Their kindness, made up for all of the years I felt unloved by the Demur's.

After burying Don, I was left settling his estate, which consisted of my childhood home and one vehicle. All of Don's money had been squandered on the horses, at the racetrack, and the house needed serious repairs. Unable to borrow enough money to fix it, I sold it to Mr. Wilson, my sister's guardian. He was a building contractor, who, after placing it on a new foundation, gave it to his son-in-law as a wedding gift. After receiving the money from the sale of the home, I moved to Virginia to buy my first restaurant. Ironically, I named it Don's Restaurant and Lounge.

Growing up in such a dysfunctional home instilled a desire within me, not to repeat the same mistakes as the Demurs. Regardless of how hard life became, I swore never to physically harm my children, abandon them or give them away to strangers. My association with the Sister's of Charity, taught me, not to hate my adoptive family. Knowing I had been a slave to them as a child, taught me not to allow them to become my masters in adulthood. Within time, I learned to forgive them completely for their mistakes. This simple and yet difficult act supernaturally released any hold they had on my life, allowing me to move forward. Now all I needed to remember was how to repeat the same act of forgiveness towards the people responsible for killing Michael, years later.

CHAPTER TWELVE

Talking with the Angels

Near-death experiences are often explained by the experts as a sensation that people on the brink of death have while leaving their bodies and observing them as though they were bystanders. Little did I know that shortly after Michael died, I would come close to losing my life and having the privilege of experiencing my first near-death experience.

During my NDE, I could see my body laying on a stretcher as the ambulance attendants working feverishly to save my life. Unaware of any time or distance, my spirit floated up high, into the clouds until Michael and I were reunited in a place called *beautiful.*

As we entered the temple, I was breathless and stood admiring the perfectly carved archways, and magnificent pillars. Since Michael was still unable to walk, I had to carry him through the temple gates. On the other side of the doorway, were six recliners placed in a circle. Somehow, I knew they were especially handcrafted for persons who could not sit unassisted. After placing him into one of the chairs, I left the area. I still can't remember where I went or why, but when I returned, Michael was gone.

I am not sure how much time lapsed before my attention was drawn towards a tall thin man, dressed in a dark suit, wearing black-framed glasses. He was standing alone next to the recliner where Michael was last seen, observing me. After asking if he had seen Michael, the spirit graciously explained that Michael was with God. Before departing, the spirit shared some encouraging news. Extending his hand towards me, I could clearly see that it held a small white piece of white parchment paper, neatly folded in two. Once opened, the words; Acts 3, verse 1-8 were clearly visible and I knew Michael was completely whole in his mind, body, and soul.

After experiencing the power of standing in *the white light*, feelings of love and understanding flooded into my being. Any fears I developed during my lifetime were removed. Following several minutes of silence, an unknown voice inquired, "What have you done with your life?" Sadly, I heard myself say; "Nothing. I have wasted the entire forty- seven years."

After choosing to return to my earthly body, I had to review all of my actions that were unkind toward others. Because of my religious upbringing, I always believed that when we die, we would be judged harshly for anything we have done wrong.

Unfortunately, I was just never sure what wrong meant. Contrary to this belief system, the light never judged me. I was made to judge myself. Another important part to my life's review demanded that I feel the same emotional pain others felt whenever I hurt their feeling with my harsh words. By seeing other people's hearts and knowing how they were affected, it caused me to feel remorseful and ashamed. Thankfully, after the experience ended, the light granted the understanding I needed and my soul found forgiveness. Before returning to earth, angels escorted me to a higher place and taught me additional lessons to share with my readers.

First, there is no such thing as time. It is man-made and self-imposed. Second, we are all brothers under the skin, and we all exist under the hood of one God. I was shown how people waste precious time fighting over what name to call God, when instead they should be acknowledging His existence and realizing that He wants nothing but the very best for us.

Third, we are all connected as one spirit. We think that we do not have any responsibility to a stranger because we do not recognize them, but we do. In essence, we are the same as they, intertwined together like a complex wiring system. This is why that old familiar phrase, *what goes around comes around* rings true. When my NDE come to an end, I understood how the different things we say in this life might injure others and how we are held accountable. Theoretically, if being cruel made another person fail to complete whatever job they were sent here to do, we will have to complete that task for them. That is why we often hear others say, "I feel like I have lived five lifetimes."

My fourth lesson was never to judge another harshly. In heaven, we get the privilege of seeing another person's heart as God would see it, we can understand how someone might react differently than we would to a particular situation. In one scene, I observed someone very standoffish. After looking into their heart, I saw how they had been injured spiritually and acted harshly out of fear. This knowledge made it easier to understand that not every action from another was about me or towards me. Sometimes it was just about them.

My final heavenly lesson taught me that all of our prayers are answered within seconds of being heard. Although it can seem like several months or years before they are answered, heaven does hear us immediately. Since time is man made and self-imposed, it does not exist in spiritual realms. In the future, anytime you need a prayer expedited in mans time, remember to recite psalms 69 and 70. Both, are our 911 to heaven!

The angel communicating with me taught me how we are 99.99% emotion and how every decision we make is based on fear. A good example would be; if we do not work, we do not eat. Reading this, you would probably agree that it is a fact of life. It is even biblical! However, the point that I am trying to make is that we do not work because it is the right thing to do and because God's Word says that we should. Most of us work out of our own fear of being hungry, homeless, or not being able to keep up with the Jones's. Consequentially, by living day to day in fear, it provides us with different motives for working and living other than the ones God has planned for us. Although attractive at first, this type of behavior can often lead to our downfall.

Once the angel took the fear factor out of the equation, I had the honor of witnessing all of the things that God had chosen for me to enjoy in this lifetime, but that I denied myself out of stubbornness. The experience helped me understand why God encourages us to place our personal feelings aside and live by trusting and believing unconditionally in Him. Before my journey ended, I knew that everything in my life happened exactly the way it was supposed to happen, when it was supposed to happen, and with whom it was supposed to happen. Confident and armed with new knowledge, I awoke in the ambulance, scaring the medics half to death!

In the end, my NDE and talking with the angels, enabled me to be at peace knowing Michael was alive and well. He shed his physical body, but his spirit was healthy and well-nourished. This experience, helped me to understand how my own fear made me act selfishly when I demanded that God allow Michael to return home with me. If I loved him, why would I ask him to live where he was misunderstood and in constant pain?

Talking with the angels taught me that I am not alone in this life. After all, Michael was just living in a different dimension until it was time for him and me to be reunited again. Having this knowledge helped me to embrace every future day with a more joyful understanding of what our life here on earth is all about, and it gave me a new form of inner peace.

CHAPTER THIRTEEN

NURSING HOME DOS AND DON'TS

Nursing home theft and abuse are quickly becoming growing concerns across the country today, and underpaid employees frequently steal items of clothing, jewelry, and money. Many times, because patients living in long-term facilities are either cognitively impaired or physically challenged, they forget what belongings are theirs. This opens the way for their possessions to become even more available to the thieves taking them. Since many states have laws that prevent a person's personal belongs from being made unavailable to them, unless it is large amounts of cash, it helps make our elderly and disabled *perfect victims*. In 1996, the *Knight-Tribune News Service* reported, "Thieves often use Vaseline to ease wedding rings off of the hands of sleeping patients. One case cited an eighty-six-year-old woman who awoke inconsolable one morning when she discovered her finger had been stripped of her life's last two mementos: a diamond ring inherited from her mother and the engagement ring her husband slipped on her finger during a romantic canoe ride. She was heartbroken!"

Often, nursing home administrators will cover up for the employee doing the stealing by either denying the theft occurred or by insisting their employees are honest, not dishonest. Because of this hear no evil, see no evil policy, police departments are hardly ever notified or asked to get involved in things so trivial as a few missing blouses or pieces of jewelry valued under one hundred dollars. If caught, employees are usually fired, but they are not made to make restitution, nor are they criminally prosecuted by either the facility or the victims' families. In July of 2001, CBS News reported a story about Helen Love, an elderly woman who was attacked by a CNA at a Sacramento, California, facility because she soiled herself.

"He choked me and went and broke my neck and broke my wrist," said Love. According to additional reports, Love's assailant received a year in the county jail. Further articles by the same newspaper revealed that three other employees employed by the same facility had been convicted for abuse as well, yet none of them was ever barred from working in any nursing facility. So why has the nursing home network ignored the need for stiffer background checks and continued to disagree that abuse has become widespread?

According to a CBS News report in 2001 and articles written in many of our national and local newspapers, most reported abuses are physical, sexual, and verbal. A congressional report written by Waxman, a top democrat on the house Government Reform Committee, which oversees spending and other operations, said he is introducing a plan that would require criminal background checks on nursing home staff and impose tougher standards on homes with violations, but where is it? Moreover, what do we call tougher standards when we allow older felons recently released from our prison system with a history of sexual assault and other violent crimes to live and work in medical facilities, so they can victimize our senior citizens and disabled children?

Why is it that congressional reports written between January 1999 and 2001 by Waxman report that over thirty percent of our nursing facilities were cited for abuse? And why were the violations serious enough to cause actual harm, immediate jeopardy of death, or serious injury? Charles H. Roadman II, president of the American Health Care Association (AHCA), a nursing home trade group that represents twelve thousand non-profit and for-profit centers and homes for the elderly and disabled, stated to CBS News in an article written on July

31, 2001, that he believes that "the great majority of long-term care in our nation is excellent." Reading articles such as these makes me wonder if any of our Congressional representatives other than Jeb Bush, have ever taken the time to visit the facilities that have been cited for these alleged abuses, or personally met with the victims screaming for justice and reform.

Whenever we seek long-term or short-term care, there are several warning signs that should never be ignored.

Below is an extensive list for the average layperson. However, when you're considering placing a family member into the hands of another, I urge you to make a copy and take it with you as you tour the facility. It may well prove to be one of the most important things you have done out of love for your disabled friend or elderly family members.

SIGNS OF PHYSICAL ABUSE:

- Not receiving immediate medical attention
- Rape
- Assault, slapping, verbal threats to hit, pinching, biting, clawing
- Black eyes, bruising, unexplained cuts, scratch marks

- Unnecessary physical restraints; being tied to a bed or chair

- No food or water.

- Improper medication/denial of medication when it is due

- Welts, red marks, swelling, mouth sores, head sores; explained and unexplained

- Restriction to chairs, rooms, or beds

- Any treatment not authorized by a physician

SIGNS OF NEGLECT:

- Inadequate access to medical personnel (nurses, doctors, medical assistants)

- Bedsores, malnutrition, dehydration

- Body odors

- Infections

- Unclean living conditions

- Failure to provide normal living conditions and services (brushing teeth, combing hair, clean underwear, etc.)

- Lack of food or water

SIGNS OF EMOTIONAL AND VERBAL ABUSE:

- Yelling or shouting at patients
- Harsh tone of voice with patients
- Irritability while dealing with patients
- Being demanding or aggressive with patients

OTHER WARNING SIGNS:

- Injuries requiring emergency procedures caused by falling out of bed/floor/showers
- Residents assaulting other residents
- Unexplained death, illness, or sudden death/illness
- Heavy sedation: excessive, unexplained sleep while visiting
- Patients missing and staff not being aware
- Broken bones, including hips
- Patients flinching or guarding their face, excessive blinking
- Patients acting anxious or afraid of their caregivers

ADDITIONAL RESOURCES

Here is a list of powerful references and outside agencies that I have provided for anyone who is interested in learning more about abuse or neglect. It will also get you started if you are interested in offering your time and services for nursing home reform. If you are not sure that someone is being abused or neglected, pay special attention to your initial instincts and report it anyway. Remember, calling local law enforcement can save a life!

1. The Centers of Medicare and Medicaid Services
   Publishes quality information about every nursing home in every state, so you know more about the services they offer.

2. Medicare Web Site
   Publishes nursing home facts, ownership, federal survey results, and populations of the nursing home you are interested in.

3. Committee on Government Reform-Minority Office. U.S. House of Representatives
   Go to the "Nursing Home Complaint Violation Search." This site lets you search for surveys based on complaints filed by other families. It will provide you with a

complete picture of the activities and care provided within the facility you are inquiring about.

4. Administration on Aging
   A federal advocate agency for older persons and their concerns. AOA works closely with its nationwide network of regional offices and state and local agencies on aging to plan, coordinate, and develop services that meet the unique needs of individual older persons and their caregivers.

5. National Citizens Coalition for Nursing Reform
   This coalition includes consumers and advocates who define and achieve quality for people with long-term care needs.

CHAPTER FOURTEEN

IN MEMORY OF MICHAEL

Nothing can be more heartbreaking than the death of a child or having to write the eulogy for a loved one, but somehow Patrick and I gathered our thoughts and tried to give Michael the best tribute we could to honor him following his passing on April 15, 1995.

Originally, there were only six people at Michael's funeral, but, after sharing this story about his life and death, I am sure there will be thousands more. If Michael were here today and could speak, he would say, "Thank you for allowing me to share my life experiences with you and for being a part of my extended family."

THE EULOGY

"In memory of Michael, I would like to offer a few words of comfort to my family and friends. Anyone who knew him or had the fortune of being in his presence, even for a moment, will always remember his laughter and his smile. He was a bright, shining star who, throughout his illness, sent a daily message full of hope and courage.

Michael was living proof that angels come in all shapes and sizes. To his family, he was their strength. He kept us together in times of adversity and hardship. He was not just a son or a brother, but a true friend to all. He was the sun on our faces, the smile on our lips, and the beat in our hearts. For his family, he taught us that *not loving* Michael meant *not loving ourselves.*

"From Christopher and Janette: "Godspeed, little brother."

"From Mom: "You were my beloved son, my best friend, and the 'wind beneath my wings.'

"As we each remember Michael in our own way, let us not mourn him in his death, but rather celebrate his new life in God's kingdom with the following Psalm:

"Blessed is he who has regard for the weak; the Lord delivers him in times of trouble. The Lord will protect him and preserve his life, he will bless him in the land and not surrender him to the desire of his foes. The Lord will sustain him on his sickbed and restore him from his bed of illness. I said "O Lord have mercy on me, heal me, for I have sinned against you." My enemies say of me in malice, "when will he die and parish?" All of my enemies whisper together against me; they imagine the worst for me saying "a vile disease has best him and he will never get up from the place where he lies." But you O' lord have mercy on me, raise me up that I may repay them. I know that you are pleased with me, for my enemy does not triumph over me. In my integrity, you uphold me and set me up in your presence forever. Praise be to the Lord, the God of Israel, from everlasting to everlasting. May He Rest In Peace! Amen and Amen."

Psalm 41, NIV

CHAPTER FIFTEEN

LADY JUSTICE

Michael's final battle with pneumonia came in March of 1995, as his body weight climbed to one hundred and twenty-five pounds. The Medicaid Waver Program we applied for was approved, and we were able to hire a caregiver, allowing Michael access to twenty-four-hour care. Unfortunately, he never lived long enough to enjoy the benefits the program offered. Along with the money for in-home services came grants for additional government programs. They provided extras like a second wheelchair ramp and construction costs for his home. Since Michael was so prone to infections, the dust from renovating the house placed him at risk. Medicaid recognized this as a real danger, so they paid for him to be moved into another retirement/assisted living community until the house was repaired. The living center we chose was a private pay or Medicare-assisted living facility. Many of the senior citizens who lived at the center loved Michael so much they treated him as a surrogate grandson.

Some, even came to his room to play cards and read him bedtime stories.

While writing this book, I remembered a humorous story about Michael and an elderly female resident, named Joan. She was his lunch companion at the assisted living center and the nursing would place their wheelchairs next to one another in the day room. Joan had long, flowing white hair that hung past her waist, and for some unknown reason Michael became fascinated by it. He also acquired an insatiable urge to touch it. It was shortly after receiving his glasses, so I am sure he saw her hair as something soft and billowy. By most accounts, Michael spent many hours wrapping his small, frail fingers around her hair, pulling it toward him. Almost daily, Joan could be heard yelling in pain, and the nurses would have to untangle her hair from Michael's fingers. Eventually, they learned to put some distance between Michael's wheelchair and Joan. However, it never deterred him. He continued trying to move his chair closer to her so he could touch her hair.

During the construction on Michael's home, several delays occurred, forcing the remodeling to be suspended for weeks at a time. Normally, that would not have been a problem, but where Michael was living was an assisted living center, and Medicaid would not pay for him to stay past the initial ninety days. Only Medicare patients or private-pay residents could stay longer. This forced us to move him back into a Medicaid nursing home.

After making several inquiries, only one nursing home in our area would accept Michael on a temporary emergency basis. When I finished touring the facility, I was concerned that it was inadequate to meet Michael's needs. The rooms were designed for double occupancy, which meant that he would have to live with an adult roommate. Another concern was that residents with Alzheimer's would wander into my son's room. Since Michael was helpless, he could not defend himself if another patient wandered into his room and tried to harm him. Unfortunately, I was not far off when I made my initial assessment regarding the facility's ability to meet Michael's needs. Two weeks after being admitted, an elderly patient living at the facility tried to suffocate my son with a pillow for the second time. According to the nursing reports, he was tired of listening to Michael laugh. The facility never reported any of the incidents to our family. They just wrote a memo and inserted it into Michael's medical file, hoping it would go unnoticed.

When Michael died, a private investigator found the memo and reported it to the nursing board and our family. Despite our outrage and repeated attempts to have the facility investigated for this and other safety violations, no action was ever taken.

One of the most common themes that seemed

to play out in Michael's life was about the time you thought you knew everything about him, something else would happen to dispel your ideas. Certainly his premature death did not put an end to his story or to what our family believed happened to him, and, as time passed, this would become even more evident. A year after Michael died, one of the caregivers who took care of him at the nursing home came to visit and shared additional details about his death. Her name was Misty, and she was on duty the night Michael died. The secret she shared with our family was horrific, and it was something that no one was privy to while his wrongful death case was being litigated. Once revealed, it would prove to be even more shocking than many of the events surrounding Michael's neglect.

On the night Michael died, his bed had been left in a downward position during his feeding, causing his stomach to overfill. As he lay begging for help, three aides and one nurse rushed into his room. After telling the aides not to start CPR, a nurse by the name of Becky left the room to get a crash cart. Instead of getting the cart, she walked to the opposite side of the hospital and met with another LPN. They began talking about a fight Becky had with her boyfriend the night before. After several minutes elapsed, Becky glanced at her watch. She was quoted as saying, "Oh, by the way, did I tell you Michael Jennings just died?"

Visibly shaken, Misty explained that Michael had died because Becky made a huge mistake when she left the head of his hospital bed flat instead of at the required thirty-degree angle. She also said that Becky "messed up bad" when she set Michael's automated feeding machine on high. Normally, it should have been set to deliver his food slowly over a six-hour period. On this particular evening, it was set to deliver his food within a few hours.

Since Michael was small for his age, setting his feeding machine on anything but low would cause his stomach to overfill, forcing his stomach contents into his lungs. Misty went on to describe Michael's death as slow and agonizing. She also stated that it was torturous for her and the other aides to watch his young life being slowly sucked away from him as they stood, doing nothing. When I asked her why she did not call 911, Misty admitted that she was afraid of losing her job. Later, when I looked through Michael's medical records, several notes supported this account of her story. One set of notes in particular, written by his pediatrician, indicated that it took over twenty minutes for him to expire. Even though it was difficult to relive the events that led up to his death, I praised Misty for having the courage to come forward.

Knowing I needed evidence to prove Michael was murdered, I asked Misty if I could record the information she provided about Becky and the other aides. Frightened that she could be implicated in a case of negligent homicide, she refused. After begging her to reconsider, I promised to talk with the authorities on her behalf. To my surprise, she relented and agreed to let me record our conversation. She said it would help alleviate her guilty conscience because she had not been able to eat or sleep since Michael died. Of course, I believed her when she said she was upset, but I also believed that she was just as responsible for the death of Michael as the charge nurse. All I needed was her confession to prove it. Armed with her confession, I drove to the attorney's office. After listening to the taped conversation, our attorney agreed that Michael died due to negligent homicide. He also promised that he would contact the district attorney's office, set up a meeting with all of the parties involved, and help our family seek criminal charges against everyone involved in Michael's death.

After the tape was placed into evidence for the wrongful death trial by our lawyer, all three nursing assistants were deposed. The tape was never used at the trial, and no one was ever held accountable for negligent homicide. Whenever our attorney tried to ask the aides about Michael's homicide, the attorney for the nursing facility self-appointed herself as their counsel and advised them not to answer any questions. Once the wrongful death case came to an end, our attorney and his paralegal disappeared, along with the majority of the money won during the lawsuit. According to the newspapers, the attorney fled to Germany to avoid any negative publicity caused from his pending divorce case. During his trial, additional allegations surfaced accusing him of laundering over thirty-plus clients' monies from other cases.

Seven years later, after working hand in hand with the Bar Association, our family finally received some justice when we learned that the attorney was disbarred from practicing law at a Supreme Court level. According to the papers, the Bar Association used our case to facilitate the charges brought against the attorney, which equaled over thirteen violations of the Standard Rules of Professional Conduct. Following the disbarment ruling, Michael's entire legal file and Misty's taped confession disappeared. The money embezzled by the lawyer was not returned, and our family was never allowed to pursue criminal charges against anyone for theft. It was considered a civil matter. Even though our family did everything possible to get justice, the police refused to file a report, and the District Attorney refused to return any of our phone calls or investigate anyone for negligent homicide.

Without revealing my sources, I can honestly say the three women who were present the night Michael died, had a history of alcoholism, drug addiction, and DUIs. As of 1998, all of them were still working in the medical field.

CONCLUSION

During the investigative phase of Michael's case, Bob Abrams, the private investigator, hired by our family presented reports from the State Board of Nursing, proving there were at least seventy-five violations filed against the nursing home where Michael died. Within the body of the report, I discovered twenty-five additional citations issued against the facility that made reference to the lack of care Michael received during his stay. Still, our family was never notified that there was a problem either by the state or the facility in question *prior* to Michael's death. In total, five additional individuals were named in the QA report. In the end, all of the people named died within one year of the initial citations being issued by the State Board of Licensing. To date, no one from the state offices, where the complaints originated, has ever taken any civil or criminal action against the people responsible for the death of Michael Jennings.

During the wrongful death negotiations, the attorneys on behalf of the insurance company and the nursing facility asked the ex-Supreme Court

Justice, who acted as mediator, to relay a message to our family. It went as follows: "We are not sorry we killed your son. As a matter of fact, Medicaid thanks us." This comment cut through our family like a knife, and it reflected the cold-blooded natures of not only our criminal justice system to allow such a vile statement, but the callous attitudes of the insurance companies that insure those facilities. Of course, I was quick to remind the Mediator, that Michael had a quality of life that was a lot richer than most people I knew. He was quick to point out that today's standards judge a person's worth based on their ability to earn a living, support a family, and pay taxes, not by who loves them.

When I was growing up, I was taught that life was precious and that we should accept it as a gift. Yet, if we listen to the legal eagles that were present at the hearing, today's standards justify the killing of disabled children or adults if they have never worked or have used Medicaid. They seemed to be trying to send a message that we as a society should support the idea that handicapped people are a liability, and it should be expected that eventually they will be disposed of. When the mediation ended, I was left knowing that money was the one deciding factor in our society that helps decide who will live and who will die. It also determines how families are compensated for the loss of a loved one.

Filing a wrongful death suit is one of the most

popular methods used to punish companies and individuals anytime there has been some form of wrongdoing. By hitting them hard in their pockets, it makes a statement loud and clear to all those who will listen. As a result, insurance companies have decided to strike back even harder by paying government officials to enact new legislation to protect the large corporation offering the minimum in health care. This act makes it almost impossible for anyone to accept responsibility for killing our children or elderly family members.

Twelve years ago, an attorney representing Michael at his wrongful death suit, knowing of the negligence and the lack of due care provided to him throughout his life, tearfully made a statement in open court regarding the care he received while in the health care system. It was profound and characterizes what I believe in my heart and soul to be true. It went as follows: "I am not surprised that Michael Jennings is dead. I am surprised that he lived as long as he did."

END NOTE

According to the legal documents filed in New Mexico, Leonard Hilton was ordered to refrain from working anywhere in or around the legal profession. He was our attorney's paralegal and the person who helped embezzled thousands of dollars from our family and other clients. When Michael's wrongful death case was mediated, Hilton requested that we sign over our insurance checks to the law office so he could deposit them into a trust account. Unfortunately, the trust account he was referring to was a dummy account set up for himself and our attorney to launder money and steal other clients' trusts. Following an indictment for embezzlement by the federal courts, Hilton fled the state to avoid prosecution. I suspect that he is still working somewhere in the law field and continuing to steal from unsuspecting clients. As I mentioned earlier, just as you think the story ends, something else appears that will shock the consciousness of every red-blooded American who will read this book. The final blow to this family's dignity came when we learned that our attorney, William Carson, was a murder suspect out of Massachusetts. When the prosecuting attorney for Alamance County could not find enough evidence to indict him, the Bar Association in Idaho gave him a license to practice law.

As Michael's story ends, my final wish is that I have been successful in showing how patients will continue to suffer as long as we as a society continue to allow power, greed, and ignorance to be the governing factors operating in our health care system. I hope that I have stirred something deep within each person who reads this book. Perhaps together we can join hands and fight for the rights of the disabled by insisting that caregivers are held accountable. Thanks to Michael, the Faith Foundation exists today. It is a non-profit organization designed to educate the public and increase public awareness regarding nursing home abuse. Please support our cause by encouraging others to read Michael's story.

May God bless!

Bibliography

Vericon News; Nursing Home Nightmare: Criminals who Care. Vol 3/Issue 1

The American Health Care Association; Report on Shortfalls in Medicaid Funding for Nursing Home Care by BDD Seidman, LLP, Accountants and Assoc.

Financial Exploitation by William Keating

Reverse Mortgages by William Keating, District Attorney of Norfolk, MA

Felons free to succeed by Doug McPherson

Texas Board of nurses examiners

Office of Economic Development; U S Work opportunity Tax Credit Program

Cerebral Palsy Help

www.cerebralplasyhelp.cpm/

March of Dimes Birth Defects Foundation
1275 Mamaroneck Avenue
White Plains, NY   10605
askus@marchofdimes.com
http://www.marchofdimes.com
Tel: 914-428-7100 888-MODIMES (663-4637)
Fax: 914-428-8203

Easter Seals
230 West Monroe Street
Suite 1800
Chicago, IL   60606-4802
info@easterseals.com
http://www.easterseals.com
Tel: 312-726-6200 800-221-6827
Fax: 312-726-1494

Children's   Neurobiological   Solutions   (CNS)
Foundation
1726 Franceschi Road
Santa Barbara, CA   93103
info@cnsfoundation.org
http://www.cnsfoundation.org
Tel: 866-CNS-5580 (267-5580) 805-965-8838

Children's Hemiplegia and Stroke Association
(CHASA)
4101 West Green Oaks Blvd., Ste. 305
PMB 149
Arlington, TX   76016

info437@chasa.org
http://www.hemi-kids.org
Tel: 817-492-4325

United Cerebral Palsy (UCP) Research & Educational
Foundation
  1660 L Street, NW
  Suite 700
  Washington, DC   20036
  national@ucp.org
  http://www.ucpresearch.org
  Tel: 202-973-7140 800-USA-5UCP (872-5827)
  Fax: 202-776-0414

CONTACT
INFORMATION:

www.brookesden.com